<u>Healthy Eating Habits</u>

A Guide to Tweaking and Balancing

the Regular Diet

(Weight Loss, Low Carb, Sugar,

Diet, Metabolism, Cravings)

By Dunstamac

herein, whether explicitly or indirectly. The copyrights not owned by the publisher belong to the writer.

The information presented here is solely for instructional purposes and is thus universal. The information is provided without some sort of guarantee or arrangement. The trademarks are used without the permission or backing of the trademark owner, and the trademark is written without the permission or backing of the trademark owner. The trademarks and labels listed in this book are the property of their respective owners, and this text is not associated with them.

Table of contents

<u>Introduction</u>

Food provides the nutrition that our bodies need to survive. Food is indeed a matter of history and custom. This may indicate that eating has an emotional aspect. Changing one's eating habits is difficult for many individuals.

You may not be aware that these food behaviors are dangerous because you have been doing them for a long time. Alternatively, your patterns have been so entrenched in your everyday routine that you don't owe them much consideration. We have a good deal of behaviors when it comes to food. Some are positive ("I always eat breakfast"), and others are negative ("I always clean my plate"). Since much of our eating patterns are formed during adolescence, it is never too late to make a shift.

With so many items and weight-loss theories on the market, it's easy to get perplexed. I've added a section on 'diet myths and reality' to help you escape a lot of the misinformation that muddles our minds around dieting and eating well. The details in this book will help to debunk misconceptions about weight loss, diet, and physical activity. Living a healthier lifestyle can become the second standard if we build improved eating habits. Learn how to eat healthily while avoiding unnecessary drama and fluff.

The jumble of good fats versus poor fats, easy meals versus slow-cooked foods, and what-to-eat and what-not-to-eat updates would undoubtedly overwhelm you in your quest to get active and balanced. The decision on whether to eat then becomes a major fight.

When it comes to healthier living, often individuals have the same challenges and concerns. You've already received contradictory reports from a variety of sources, and you now believe you have no idea what good eating entails. Then you start asking yourself a lot of questions.

This book will show you...

- The significance of a balanced diet

- Taking care of your eating in the proper manner

- How to correctly search for nutritious foods

- When do you take supplements?

- How to eat healthily without relying on menus or complicated instructions

- Maintain a safe lifestyle even though you're out and about or on vacation.

- Ingenious strategies to get the kids to consume nutritious meals

In this book, some bad eating habits are discussed with detailed solutions. In the pages below some healthy foods, habits, and strategies are discussed, these will definitely help you to return to a healthy lifestyle. You'll be motivated to make smarter decisions and live your life to the fullest extent possible.

Chapter 1.   Eating Habits

Eating habits (also known as dietary habits) relate to when and how individuals consume, what foods they eat, and from whom they eat, as well as how they receive, store, use, and dump food. Individuals' eating habits are influenced by a variety of variables including social, cultural, religious, fiscal, environmental, and political factors.

Why and How People Eat?

Humans must feed in order to live. They even eat to show gratitude, to feel a sense of belonging, to follow family traditions, and to achieve self-realization. Someone who is not hungry, for example, may eat a slice of cake baked in his or her honor.

People eat according to etiquette, meal and snack patterns, acceptable foods, food combinations, and portion sizes that they have learned. Acceptable behaviors are referred to as etiquette. For example, some cultures consider it acceptable to lick one's fingers while eating, while others consider it impolite. Depending on whether the meal is formal, informal, or special, etiquette and eating rituals differ (such as a meal on a birthday or religious holiday).

A meal is typically defined as the consumption of two or more foods at a predetermined time in a structured setting. Snacks are small portions of food or beverages consumed in between meals. Three meals (breakfast, lunch, and dinner) per day, with snacks in between, is a common eating pattern. A meal's components vary by culture, but they typically include grains like rice or noodles, meat or a meat substitute like fish, beans, or tofu, and side dishes like vegetables. Various food guides offer advice on what to eat, how much to eat, and how much to drink on a daily basis. Personal preferences, habits, family customs, and social setting, on the other hand, heavily influence what a person consumes.

What do people eat?

There are acceptable and unacceptable foods in every culture, but this is not determined by whether or not something is edible. Alligators, for example, are found in many parts of the world, but many people refuse to eat them. Horses, turtles, and dogs, for example, are eaten (and even considered delicacies) in some cultures but are not acceptable food sources in others. There are also rules about who it is acceptable to eat with. Doctors in a healthy hospital, for example, can eat in different areas from patients or customers.

Getting, Preserving, Consuming, and Tossing Away Food

Food is obtained, preserved, and discarded in a number of forms by humans. Any food is grown, fished, or hunted, while the majority is purchased from supermarkets or specialized stores. People can store small amounts of food and get the majority of what they eat on a daily basis if they have limited access to energy sources. People who live in houses with plenty of room and electricity, on the other hand, buy food in bulk and store it in freezers, refrigerators, and pantries. In any scenario, appropriate disposal facilities are needed to prevent environmental and health issues.

Exposure to Food

There are a plethora of spices and cuisine varieties to choose from. Some tastes or food blends are easy to consider, whereas others must be developed or studied. Sweetness is widely liked, but a palate for salty, savory, spicy, sour, bitter, and hot flavors must be created. The more a human is introduced to food and motivated to consume it, the more likely they are to consider it. If a person's sensitivity to food rises, they become more comfortable with it and less afraid of it, and approval may grow. Some people consume only such foods and flavor blends, while others enjoy experimenting with new foods and tastes.

Chapter 2.   Influences on Food Choices

There are numerous factors that influence what food an individual eats. There are cultural, social, religious, technological, environmental, and even political considerations in addition to personal interests.

2.1.   Individual Preferences

When it comes to cooking, everybody has their own tastes. Personal interactions such as motivation to consume, introduction to a diet, family customs and traditions, advertisement, and personal beliefs all affect these habits over time. For example, despite the fact that frankfurters are a family tradition, one individual may dislike them.

2.2.   Cultural Influences

Appropriate items, food combinations, eating habits, and eating practices are all described by a cultural community. Individuals that follow these rules develop a sense of self-identity and belonging. Subgroups occur within broad ethnic groups that may follow variants of the larger group's eating habits while also being deemed a member of the larger group. An average American meal, for example, consists of a hamburger, French fries, and a beer. In the United States, though, vegetarians consume "veggie-burgers" made from mashed beans, pureed tomatoes, or soy, and dieters may eat a lean turkey burger. There are acceptable cultural substitutions in the United States, but a horsemeat burger will be unethical.

2.3. Social Influences

A social group's members are reliant on one another, share a shared community, and affect one another's attitudes and beliefs. Food habits are influenced by a person's participation in specific peer, career, or neighborhood groups. For example, at a basketball game, a young person might consume some foods with his or her friends and other foods with his or her instructor.

2.4. Religious influences

The number of religious prohibitions varies greatly, from a few to a large number, and from casual to rigid. And would have an effect on a follower's eating habits and attitudes. For example, some items are forbidden in certain sects, such as pork among Jewish and Muslim followers. Under Christianity, Seventh-day Adventists discourage the use of "stimulating" drinks such as beer, which is not prohibited by Catholics.

2.5. Economic Influences

What an individual buys, is influenced by money, beliefs, and customer skills. The cost of a meal, on the other hand, is not a reliable measure of its nutritional value. The cost of food is calculated by a dynamic mixture of its supply, status, and demand.

2.6. Environmental Influences

The climate has an effect on eating patterns due to a combination of ecological and social influences. Foods that are widely available and easy to grow in a particular area often become part of the local cuisine. Many foods that were formerly only accessible during those seasons or in certain areas are now available virtually everywhere, at any time, thanks to new technologies, farming techniques, and transportation methods.

2.7. Political Influences

Food supply and patterns are often affected by political influences. Food policies and trade deals have an effect on what is accessible inside and across nations, as well as on food costs. Consumers' awareness of the food they buy is determined by food labeling rules.

Eating patterns are thus influenced by both external and internal influences, such as politics and morals. These patterns are developed over a person's lifespan and can alter.

Chapter 3. Diet and Nutrition

3.1.   Bad Eating Habits and How to Break Them

Snacking late at night, emotional feeding, and junk-food binges ring a bell? Breaking these typical poor eating patterns will help you lose weight quickly.

Overeating and weight gain were caused by more than just a loss of motivation. It's also the sly poor habit you picked up without even noticing it, like rushing out the door without eating some mornings or munching chips while watching your favorite TV program. The next thing you know, one little poor behavior has added up to a large amount of weight gain. Worst of all, you might not even be aware of what you're doing to your diet.

Here are several fast remedies for some of the more popular dietary and lifestyle patterns that can lead to weight gain.

3.1.1. The Bad Habit: Mindless Eating

Brian Wansink, Ph.D., a Cornell University food psychologist, found that the bigger the plate or cup you feed on, the more you unconsciously drink. Wansink discovered in a recent survey that moviegoers who were provided extra-large containers of expired popcorn nevertheless consumed 45 percent more than those who ate fresh popcorn from smaller containers containing the same number.

The Solution: Consume food from smaller plates. Try using a salad plate instead of a big dinner plate, and never feed directly from a cup or box.

3.1.2.   The Bad Habit: Eating Late at Night

According to diet folklore, feeding late at night is almost never a smart thing if you're trying to lose weight. Despite the fact that many scientists assume this old adage is a fallacy, a recent animal report reinforces the notion that it's not only what you consume, but even what you eat that matters. Mice fed high-fat diets throughout the day (when these nocturnal animals could have been sleeping) gained slightly more weight than mice fed the same diet at night, according to Northwestern University researchers.

The Solution: Is this a diet take-out joint? After dinner, tell yourself that the kitchen is locked for the night and brush your teeth — a freshly washed mouth may make you want to eat less. Wait 10 minutes if you have a craving. If you're ever hungry, take a quick snack such as string cheese or a slice of fruit.

3.1.3. The Bad Habit: Excessive Snacking

Snacking around the clock, mostly on high-calorie snacks high in empty carbohydrates, is a terrible habit that many people have. It's not just a challenge for adults, according to a new survey from the University of North Carolina: kids are snacking more and more on unhealthy fast food like fatty snacks, soda, and sweets.

According to Jessica Crandall, RD, a spokesperson for the American Dietetic Association, hold only nutritious snacks within scopes, such as hummus, carrots and cucumber sticks, air-popped popcorn, milk, and almonds. Don't have potato chips or treats on your desk or in your pantry that you know you'll eat.

3.1.4. The Bad Habit: Skipping Breakfast

You realize that breakfast is the most important meal of the day, however, you may decide that you don't have time to eat because you have too many other things to do. When you miss meals, your metabolism slows down, according to Crandall, and breakfast offers you the injection of energy you need to get through the day. You'll definitely overeat later if you don't have this power. Over a two-year stretch, Chinese schoolchildren who missed breakfast gained slightly more weight than those who consumed a morning meal, according to a new report.

The Solution: Get nutritious breakfast snacks on hand so you can eat on the go, according to Crandall. If you're short of time, go for simple foods like whole berries, milk, homemade cereal bars, and smoothies.

3.1.5. The Bad Habit: Emotional Eating

You've had a tough day at work, but when you get home, you open the refrigerator and consume something unhealthy — not a smart eating plan. Crandall explains, "You bring food in your mouth as a calming mechanism." A variety of studies show that people's feelings, both good and negative, may encourage them to consume more than they should, which is a common weight-loss roadblock.

The Solution: According to Crandall, is to discover a different stress reliever. "If you're stressed out at college, go for a stroll instead of eating or call a sympathetic buddy when you get home "she proposes "You will let off steam and relieve some of the stress." You can do anything you want as long as it takes you away from the kitchen.

3.1.6. The Bad Habit: Eating too Fast

If you're snacking or enjoying a meal, wolfing down the food doesn't allow your head time to catch up with your stomach. It takes 15 to 20 minutes for your brain to register that you're complete once you've stopped feeding. If you consume your meal in less than 10 minutes, you can consume much more than you need. Japanese researchers discovered that consuming very fast was closely linked to becoming overweight in a survey of 3,200 men and women.

The Solution: To eat more slowly, place your fork down between bites, take smaller bites, and chew each bite thoroughly. Additionally, consuming water after the meal can assist you in slowing down and feeling fuller.

3.1.7. The Bad Habit: Not Getting Enough Sleep

Is it possible that not having enough sleep would sabotage the weight-loss efforts? Yes, according to a new study conducted by Tokyo researchers. Men and women who slept five hours or less a night were shown to be more likely to gain weight than someone who slept seven hours or more a night.

The Solution: Establish a daily schedule for yourself, and aim to go to bed and wake up at the same time every day, except on weekends. Keep the space quiet and warm, and stop watching TV or using laptops for at least an hour before heading to bed. If you need more inspiration to go to bed early, keep in mind that the better you sleep, the better the number on the scale would be in the morning.

3.1.8.   The Bad Habit: Vegging Out with Video Games

Whether you're watching TV, seated in front of a monitor, or playing video games, you don't just have to think about mindless snacking in front of the television. According to a recent survey, teenagers who spent one-hour playing video games consumed more the remainder of the day, resulting in weight gain. The researchers aren't exactly why boys who play video games consume more, although they believe that sitting in front of a screen all day could have a similar impact on adults, leading to snacking.

The Solution: Take regular breaks from the screen — 45 to 60 minutes, get up, and move around the space or workplace. When the workday or your favorite TV program is done, try to keep track of what you eat so you don't overeat.

3.1.9. The Bad Habit: Eating Junk Food

You may realize that fast food is bad for your waistline, but the result might be much greater. Several experimental experiments also discovered that high-fat, high-sugar diets are toxic to rats' brains, comparable to cocaine or heroin. Another research discovered that consuming comfort food really makes people feel happy.

The Solution: According to research, excluding your favorite indulgences from your diet would just help you miss them more. The trick to weight reduction success is to figure out what you really desire and only enjoy it in the balance as unique treats rather than every day.

<u>Chapter 4.   Eat well</u>

The trick to a healthier diet is to obtain the appropriate number of calories for your level of activity so that the nutrition you take is balanced with the energy you expend. You can accumulate weight if you eat unhealthily or consume more than the body requires and the nutrition you cannot use is retained as fat. You can lose weight if you eat and drink too little. You can also eat a number of foods to guarantee that you have a well-balanced diet and that the body is having all of the nutrients it needs.

Men can eat roughly 2,500 calories a day (10,500 kilojoules). A woman's daily calorie intake should be about 2,000 calories (8,400 kilojoules). The majority of adults in the United Kingdom consume more calories than they require and can consume fewer calories.

4.1. Useful tips to eat well

These eight useful tips cover the foundations of safe eating and will assist you in making smart decisions.

4.1.1. Eat more high-fiber starchy carbs

Just over a portion of your diet can be made up of starchy carbohydrates. Potatoes, bread, rice, noodles, and cereals are among them. Choose wholewheat spaghetti, brown rice, or potatoes with their skins on for higher fiber or wholegrain types.

They have more fiber than white or processed starchy carbs, but they will keep you feeling fuller much longer. With each main meal, try to provide at least one starchy food. Some people believe starchy foods are fattening, but the carbohydrate they produce contains less than half the calories of a fat gram.

When frying or serving these things, keep an eye on the fats you use because this is what lifts the calorie count – for example, oil on chips, butter on toast, and creamy sauces on pasta.

4.1.2. Consume a variety of fruits and vegetables

Every day, you can consume at least 5 portions of a number of fruits and vegetables. They come in a range of ways, including raw, frozen, bottled, dry, and juiced. Having that 5 A Day is not as complicated as it may seem. Replace your midmorning snack with a slice of fresh fruit by chopping a banana over your breakfast cereal.

80g is a serving of natural, dried, or frozen fruit and vegetables. 30g of dried fruit (which can be served mainly at mealtimes). A 150ml glass of fruit juice, vegetable juice, or smoothie counts as one serving, just restrict yourself to one glass per day since these beverages are rich in sugar and will damage your teeth.

4.1.3.   Increase the seafood consumption, including a part of fatty fish

Fish is high in calcium and includes a variety of vitamins and minerals. Aim to consume at least two servings of fish each week, each of which should be oily.

Omega-3 fats found in oily fish can help to prevent heart disease.

Fish that are high in oil include:

- Salmon

- trout

- herring

- sardines

- pilchards

- mackerel

Fish that aren't oily include:

- haddock

- plaice

- coley

- cod

- tuna

- skate

- hake

Note: New, frozen, and packaged fish are all options, but canned and smoked fish include a lot of salt. While most people can consume more fish, certain varieties of fish have proposed restrictions.

4.1.4. Minimize the amount of saturated fat and sugar in the diet

Saturated fat is an unhealthy kind of fat. You need fat in your diet, but the quantity and form of fat you consume must be carefully monitored. Saturated and unsaturated fats are the two major categories of fat. Over much-saturated fat in your diet will raise your blood cholesterol levels, increasing your risk of heart disease.

Note: Men can consume no more than 30 grams of saturated fat a day on average. Women can eat no more than 20 grams of saturated fat a day on average.

Kids under the age of 11 should consume fewer saturated fat than adults, but children under the age of 5 should not consume a low-fat diet.

Saturated fat can be present in a number of foods, including:

- fatty cuts of meat

- sausages

- butter

- hard cheese

- cream

- cakes

- biscuits

- lard

- pies

Reduce the consumption of saturated fats and replace them with unsaturated fats from things like edible oils and spreads, fatty fish, and avocados. Using a small amount of vegetable or olive oil, or a reduced-fat spread instead of butter, lard, or ghee for a healthy substitute. When eating meat, choose lean cuts and trim away any noticeable fat. Since all forms of fat are rich in calories, they should be consumed in moderation.

4.1.5. Sugar

Eating high-sugar foods and beverages on a daily basis increases the chance of obesity and tooth loss. Sugary foods and beverages are rich in energy (measured in kilojoules or calories) and can lead to weight gain if drunk too often. They may also induce tooth decay if consumed in between meals.

Sugars applied to foods or beverages, as well as sugars contained naturally in butter, syrups, and unsweetened fruit juices and smoothies, are also examples of free sugars. Rather than the sugar present in fruits and milk, this is the kind of sugar you should be avoiding. Free sugars are present in surprising quantities in many foods and beverages.

Free sugars can be present in a variety of foods, including:

- sugary fizzy drinks

- sugary breakfast cereals

- cakes

- biscuits

- pastries and puddings

- sweets and chocolate

- alcoholic drinks

Food labeling may be useful. Use them to determine how much sugar is in foods. Food with more than 22.5g of total sugars per 100g is heavy in sugar, whereas food with less than 5g of total sugars per 100g is poor in sugar. Learn how to reduce the amount of sugar in your diet.

4.1.6. Limit the salt intake to no more than 6 grams a day for adults

Too much salt in your diet will increase your blood pressure. High blood pressure makes you more likely to have heart problems or experience a stroke. You could be consuming too much even though you don't add salt to your diet.

Around three-quarters of the salt, you ingest is already found in items such as breakfast cereals, soups, bread, and sauces before you purchase them.

To help you save from salts, look at product labeling. The presence of more than 1.5g of salt per 100g suggests that the food is salty. Adults and children aged 11 and up can consume no more than 6g (approximately a teaspoonful) of salt a day. Kids under the age of six can have much fewer.

4.1.7. Keep exercising and sustain a healthier weight.

Daily exercise, in addition to eating healthily, can help lower your risk of developing serious health problems. It's also crucial for good fitness and happiness.

Type 2 diabetes, some tumors, cardiac failure, and stroke may also be caused by being overweight or obese. Being underweight will have a detrimental effect on your well-being. Most people need to reduce their calorie intake in order to lose weight.

If you wish to lose weight, strive to eat less and do more. Maintaining a good weight may be as easy as consuming a healthy, nutritious diet. Use the BMI balanced weight calculator to see whether you're at a healthy weight. Begin the NHS weight-loss program, a 12-week plan that incorporates a balanced diet with physical exercise guidance. See underweight adults if you're underweight. If you're nervous about your weight, contact your doctor or a dietitian.

4.1.8. Do not get thirsty

To avoid being dehydrated, you can consume lots of water. The government advises that you consume 6 to 8 glasses of water a day. This is in comparison to the fluid you ingest from your food.

Both non-alcoholic beverages are appropriate, but water, low-fat milk, and low-sugar beverages, such as tea and coffee, are better alternatives. Sugary soft and fizzy beverages are rich in calories, so skip them. They're even detrimental to your dental health. Free sugar is included in still unsweetened fruit juice and smoothies.

Your regular total of beverages including fruit juice, vegetable juice, and smoothies does not reach 150ml, which is around half a bottle. If it's sunny outside or you're running, try to take some water.

4.1.9. Do not skip breakfast

Some people say missing breakfast can help them lose weight. A nutritious breakfast rich in fiber and low in calories, sugar, and salt, on the other hand, will help you get the nutrients you need for good health as part of a regular diet. A delicious and healthier breakfast is whole grain lower-sugar cereal with semi-skimmed milk and fruit slices on top.

<u>Conclusion</u>

This book "Healthy Eating Habits" will assist you in achieving a healthy lifestyle. Often, think of the good behaviors you already have and be aware of them. Learn not to be overly hard on yourself when it comes to your acts. It's quick to get caught up in your bad habits. This will cause you to get stressed and give up on your efforts to improve.

The first meal of the day sets the pace for the rest of the day. A filling, balanced meal can supply the body with the resources it takes to bring you to lunch. If you're not hungry when you wake up, a glass of milk or small fruit and dairy-based smoothie may be a decent choice. We also have exercise and diet aspirations when it comes to our well-being, such as gaining weight, exercising more, eating healthy, or making smart food decisions. It might take months to lose weight. Daily exercise may take years, although eating healthy and making informed dietary decisions are impossible to calculate. We will become frustrated and give up before achieving these objectives. To keep on track, we should break down our fitness objectives into simpler, more achievable measures - steps that are easy to calculate and track weekly or monthly so we can see our success and stay inspired.

If you find yourself resuming an old routine, consider why you did so. Replace that with a fresh habit once more. You are not a loser because you made a mistake. Continue to pursue!